TABLE OF CONTENTS

IF YOUR CHILD IS OVERWEIGHT

A Guide for Parents

Fourth Edition

Susan M. Kosharek, MS, RD

Academy of Nutrition and Dietetics
Chicago, IL

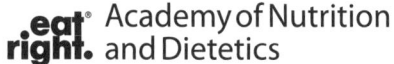

eat® Academy of Nutrition
right. and Dietetics

If Your Child is Overweight: A Guide for Parents, Fourth Edition

ISBN 978-0-88091-990-6

Catalog Number 303717

The views expressed in this publication are those of the authors and do not necessarily reflect policies and/or official positions of the Academy of Nutrition and Dietetics. Mention of product names in this publication does not constitute endorsement by the authors or the Academy of Nutrition and Dietetics. The Academy of Nutrition and Dietetics disclaims responsibility for the application of the information contained herein.

10   9   8   7   6   5   4   3   2   1

For more information on the Academy of Nutrition and Dietetics, visit www.eatright.org.

INTRODUCTION

If you are unsure how to help your overweight child, becoming well informed is a good place to start. As a parent or caregiver, having the right information can help a child reach and maintain a healthy weight.

When children gain too much weight, this can increase their risk for:

- diabetes and other diseases, such as cancer, heart disease, high blood pressure, high cholesterol and triglycerides (fats in the blood), and stroke;

- breathing problems like sleep apnea or asthma;

- being obese as adults; and

- developing bone and joint problems.

In addition to these health problems, being overweight can cause emotional pain too. Children who are overweight may be discriminated against, or they may feel isolated.

It's clear there are many risks for children who are overweight. However, it's important to know that the ways that adults lose weight are usually not right for children. Children are growing and developing. Therefore, they have special nutritional needs. A diet that is too limited may keep children from growing and developing as they should.

This booklet is written for parents with overweight children between the ages of 4 and 12 years. It explains what you need to know about your child's nutritional and growth needs, and it shows ways to improve the eating habits of your entire family. By changing the way your whole family eats, it will be easier for your overweight child to maintain healthy eating habits.

IS MY CHILD OVERWEIGHT?

Parents often use standards meant for adults to evaluate the weight and body shape of their children. But this is a mistake. Children have different weight standards and body shapes than adults. Also, as children develop, the amount of body fat that they need to be healthy will change. And while children usually gain weight at a fairly steady rate, at times they may gain weight quickly, such as just before a growth spurt.

For these reasons, it can be hard to correctly evaluate your child's weight yourself. However, a doctor or a registered dietitian nutritionist (RDN) can find your child's healthy weight range. Doctors and RDNs use tools such as body mass index (BMI) and growth charts to track children's growth patterns. They may also check a child's bone size, body type, and amount of muscle. All of these factors help them decide the healthy weight range for each child.

Body Mass Index

BMI is a way of measuring heaviness using your child's height and weight. A doctor may use it to follow your child's body size over time. If you don't already know your child's BMI, you can use Box 1 to calculate it.

BOX 1 Calculating Body Mass Index

$$BMI = \frac{Weight\ (in\ pounds)}{[Height\ (in\ inches) \times Height\ (in\ inches)]} \times 703$$

For example: To find the BMI for a child who weighs 102 pounds and is 58 inches tall:

$$BMI = \frac{102}{58 \times 58} \times 703 = 21.3$$

Your child's doctor can analyze this number by plotting it on a BMI-for-age chart, which looks similar to the growth chart that is used to track how a child grows. Separate BMI charts are used for boys and girls. The doctor may then tell you that your child's BMI is at a certain *percentile*. The percentile shows how your child's BMI compares to boys or girls of the same age. Using the BMI percentile, a doctor or RDN can interpret the results to assess your child's weight status as follows:

BMI Percentile Range	Weight Category
Less than the 5th Percentile	Underweight
5th to 84th Percentile	Normal or Healthy weight
85th to 94th Percentile	Overweight
95th percentile or greater	Obese

The percentile does not measure body fat directly, but it shows where your child falls in relation to other children of the same age. For example, if a 10-year-old boy has a BMI at the 90th percentile, it would mean his body size is greater than 90% of boys his age. For an online tool that calculates your child's BMI and percentile, go to: nccd.cdc. gov/dnpabmi/calculator.aspx.

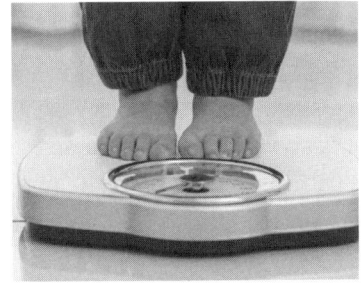

Keep in mind that BMI is not a perfect tool, and a single measurement is not enough. A high BMI is a signal that your child may have a weight problem. If your child is very muscular or has a large frame size, he or she may have a high BMI but not be overweight. It's also important to look at family history, eating habits, and the amount of physical activity your child gets.

However, BMI can be very helpful for identifying children who are at risk of becoming overweight. It's important to measure BMI at least once per year, or more often if your doctor recommends it, to decide whether a child's weight is increasing too quickly. For example, if a child's BMI is around the 35th percentile but then jumps up to the 65th percentile in 6 to 12 months, his or her doctor will want to check this out.

The change may be due to normal growth and weight gain during puberty. Or there may be some other reason for the weight gain. A doctor can decide whether something in your child's lifestyle should be changed to help control his or her weight.

The doctor will keep track of your child's BMI over time. If there are any trends or sudden changes that need to be addressed, the doctor will discuss this with you. Together you can plan a course of action, which may include working with an RDN to help your child learn and practice healthy weight habits.

What Is Normal Growth?

Children grow at different speeds at different times. Before puberty, they grow at a pretty regular pace. Each year, they get about two inches taller and gain about 5 to 10 pounds. It is normal for their BMI to change during this time. It is also normal for children under age 7 or 8 to have some "baby fat." They should lose this when they hit a growth spurt.

About two years into puberty, children grow more quickly. At this time, a child can grow 4 to 6 inches in less than a year. During this growth spurt, many children gain more body fat. This kind of weight gain is especially common in girls. It is normal weight gain also known as prepubescent growth. In girls, it may begin by age 7 or 8. In boys, it begins around age 9 or 10. About 50 percent of children reach it by age 11. The growth spurt usually lasts about 18 to 24 months. However, it may last several years.

When children grow quickly, they need more nutrients and calories. For this reason, dieting and weight loss are not recommended for most children. However, with careful planning, eating habits can be adjusted so that before puberty, overweight children stay at the same weight or lose weight very slowly. Then, as children hit the adolescent growth spurt, their weight may be right for their new height.

Risk Factors for Weight Gain

If your child is not currently considered overweight but you are worried about his or her lifestyle and eating habits, take a look at Box 2. How many of these points describe your child? If just one or two of the items are true for your child, that's okay. But if more points apply, then he or she may be more likely to gain extra weight.

BOX 2 **Possible Causes for Weight Gain**

Gets little physical activity (less than 60 minutes per day)

Snacks frequently on high-fat and high-calorie foods, such as chips, cookies, candy, crackers, and ice cream

Does not eat at regular mealtimes every day

Skips meals and snacks throughout the day

Has overweight family members

Watches two or more hours of TV daily

Has access to a TV in dining room or bedroom

Spends several hours each day using the computer or playing video games

Snacks while watching TV or playing video games

Eats a lot of sugary or fried foods

Eats fast food more than once per week

Drinks sweetened beverages daily—for example, soda, juice drinks, fruit juice, and highly sweetened milk drinks

Is taller than other kids his or her age

Gets less than 8 hours of sleep each night

Eats increased portion sizes

WHY IS MY CHILD OVERWEIGHT?

Many factors contribute to weight problems in children. A tendency to be overweight runs in families. However, this does not mean that a child with overweight parents is sure to be overweight. Heredity is just one part of the picture.

Family patterns such as eating and activity habits may have a much stronger influence on weight than genetics. These habits are considered environmental factors. Emotional factors may also play a role.

Environmental Factors

Many things in a person's environment can lead to weight gain. For example:

- The type and amount of food available

- Activity level

- Snacking habits

- Using food for reward or punishment

- Amount of time spent watching TV, using the computer, and playing video games

- Eating at restaurants or fast food places more than once a week

- Drinking lots of sugar-sweetened beverages

There are many things you can do to change these environmental factors. For example, help your child to be active every day. Limit total time in front of the screen to one or two hours per day. Have your child get up and move around during commercials. Encourage your child to do other activities—watching TV burns about 50 calories per hour, but playing tag burns about 500 calories per hour.

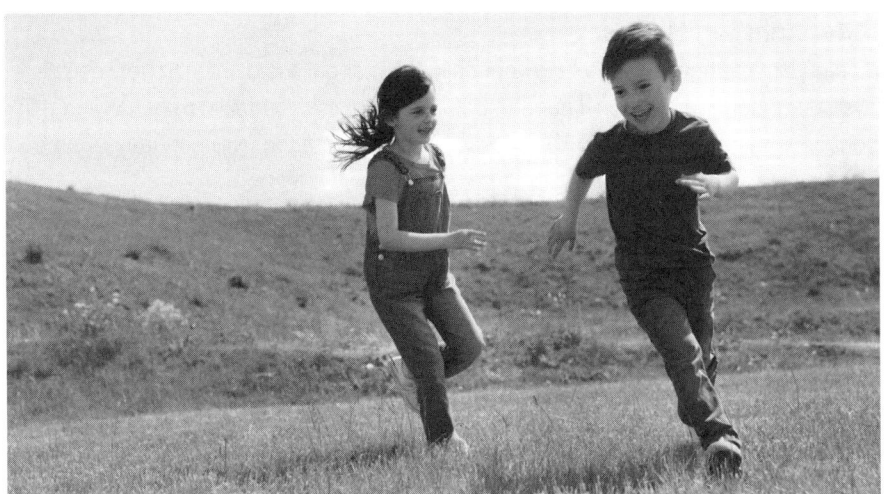

Also consider having a family rule against eating while watching TV, using the computer, or playing video games. Many children mindlessly snack on high-calorie foods, such as crackers, chips, and cookies, while they watch TV or play computer games. They might not even be aware of how much they are eating!

Some medicines may increase weight gain or appetite. Check with your child's doctor about this. Maybe your child can take different medicines.

Emotional Factors

There are two basic types of hunger: emotional and physical. Emotional hunger means eating to deal with feelings. Physical hunger is the body's signal that it needs energy and nutrients. It's okay for children to feel both types of hunger, but if they get used to eating when they feel emotional hunger, they may end up relying on food to avoid strong feelings that can be uncomfortable or hard to handle. Children who say they are always hungry may be eating for emotional reasons.

If your child eats as a way of dealing with feelings, he or she can forget what physical hunger feels like. If you think that your child is overeating for emotional reasons, help him or her learn how to deal with his or her feelings in a healthy way. Remind your child that emotions are normal, but food can't solve problems. Food may make problems seem better for a little while, but the problems are still there. Talk to your child's doctor or a RDN. They can help you find out what may be going on with your child and may be able to suggest healthier ways for your child to cope.

Understanding Hunger

You can use a hunger scale to help your child learn about the difference between physical hunger and emotional hunger. Before eating, ask your child to pause and think about how he or she is feeling. Then ask your child to rate the feeling of hunger on a scale from 1 to 10:

Hunger Scale

Very Hungry	Hungry	Not Hungry or Full	Full	Stuffed
1	3	5	7	10

● ●

- 1 means you are very, very hungry, and you might feel lightheaded, irritable

- 5 means you are neither hungry nor full and feel satisfied

- 10 means you feel completely stuffed, so full you might feel sick

After using the hunger scale for a while, it will be easier for your child to rate his or her feelings of hunger. It can take a while to truly know what a high or low number feels like. Once you are both familiar with the scale, it can help your child learn when to start and stop eating.

The basic idea is to start eating when hunger is at a 2 or 3. At this point, your child is eating because of physical hunger. Ask your child to stop eating when he or she reaches around a 6 or 7 on the scale. At this point, your child should feel satisfied but not overstuffed. Try not to let your child's hunger level drop to a 1. If your child gets this hungry, he or she may overeat.

If a child starts to eat when the score on the hunger scale is above a 5, he or she is probably eating for emotional reasons. Take this opportunity to discover which feelings are behind the desire to eat. If your child has this type of hunger, you may help him or her by asking, "How do you feel?" Your child may have trouble naming his or her feelings, and that's okay. You can help out by suggesting a few. (Box 3 lists some common feelings.)

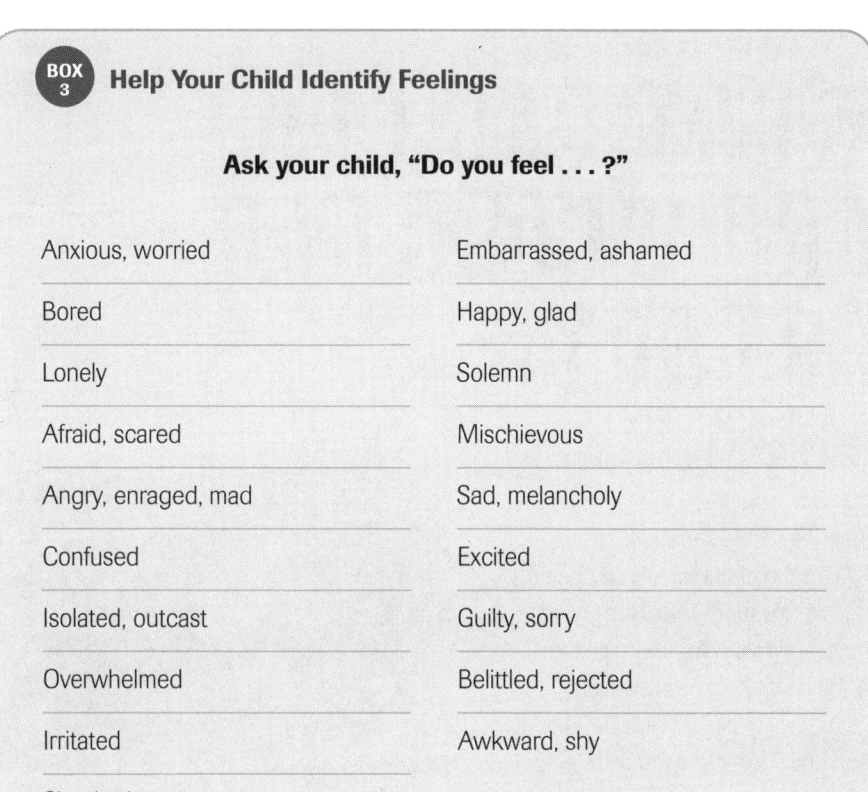

BOX 3 — Help Your Child Identify Feelings

Ask your child, "Do you feel . . . ?"

Anxious, worried	Embarrassed, ashamed
Bored	Happy, glad
Lonely	Solemn
Afraid, scared	Mischievous
Angry, enraged, mad	Sad, melancholy
Confused	Excited
Isolated, outcast	Guilty, sorry
Overwhelmed	Belittled, rejected
Irritated	Awkward, shy
Shocked	

If your child can tell you about his or her feelings, this may be a good time to talk. You can also encourage older children to write in a journal about their feelings if they feel uncomfortable talking about them out loud.

In order to combat emotional hunger, once you identify the emotions behind eating, perhaps you and your child can think of other activities to do that do not involve food. For example, if a child feels left out, maybe you can talk or play a game together. Or if your child is angry about something, maybe you can brainstorm ways to work on the problem.

WHAT CAN I DO AND WHERE CAN I START?

You are your child's role model! Kids are more likely to make lifestyle changes if they see their parents making the changes first. By being a good role model, you are laying the groundwork for your child to develop life-long healthy eating habits, which are more important than any short-term diet.

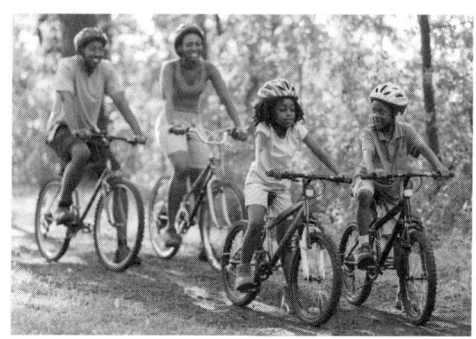

Get the whole family involved.
Everyone will learn healthy habits, and the overweight child will not feel singled out.

Be Supportive, Not Controlling

Try not to treat your child differently because of his or her weight. Treat your child as you would if he or she were not overweight.

Let your child know that he or she is okay whatever he or she weighs. Provide him or her with a healthy environment that includes plenty of activity and healthy foods, and try playing fun active games together. Try to make being active fun rather than forcing your child to be active, which might make it seem like a chore.

Do not control the amount of food your child eats. This may lead your child to think too much about food, and then he or she may overeat. A strict diet might also send the message to your child that you are not happy with his or her size, and your child might view it as rejection, thinking that you will love your child more when he or she is thinner. Your child needs to decide how much to eat. Your job is to make sure that there are plenty of healthy foods to choose from.

Talk with Your Child

Go ahead and talk with your child about weight. Allow your child to tell you about feelings that he or she may not have talked about before. Your child may be teased at school. Maybe your child doesn't do well in sports. Maybe your child is usually chosen last for teams. Or maybe your child is embarrassed because he or she has trouble fitting into his or her clothes. These frustrating and painful issues are common among overweight children.

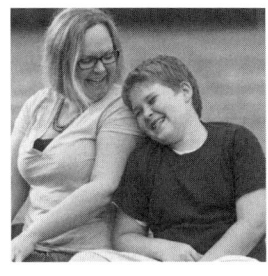

If your child shares these feelings with you, listen to your child. Let your child know that his or her feelings are real, frustrating, and painful. If you have had similar experiences, it may help to share them. You can use this as an opportunity to explain that people come in all different sizes and shapes and to reassure your child that you will accept him or her and love your children no matter what their size. Overweight children need support, acceptance, reassurance, and encouragement from their parents.

Encourage your child to share his or her feelings whenever they arise. Let your child know that you will listen when he or she needs to talk. However, never force your child to talk about anything he or she is not ready to discuss.

Set Realistic Goals

Remember that the main goal for your overweight child may be to slow the rate of weight gain. Or the goal may be for your child to stay at his or her current weight while he or she grows taller.

Based on these goals, it may take 6 months or longer for your child to grow into his or her weight. The amount of time will depend on your child's weight and when his or her growth spurts take place.

When setting goals, it is important to:

- **Realize that change occurs slowly.** Be patient. It can be hard to change eating habits. Aim for what is possible, not for perfection.

- **Change menus slowly.** Try one new dish or type of food at a time. If your family is used to fast food, they may not be ready for a menu of chicken breast and baked potatoes or broiled fish and carrots.

- **Set yourself up for success.** Choose a few specific changes that you can make. Use the Family Lifestyle Quiz (page 13) to find changes you can make in your family's eating habits.

- **Make weekly goals and track progress.** Set up a family goal contract with your family (see sample below). For example, you could set a goal to have fresh fruit at every meal for a week. Write that goal down. Then mark off every day or every meal that you meet it. You don't need to be perfect. If you hit the goal most of the time, that's great. Set goals every week until you feel you have made lasting changes that promote a healthy lifestyle. Reward your family with nonfood prizes, such as a trip to the movies or a bowling outing.

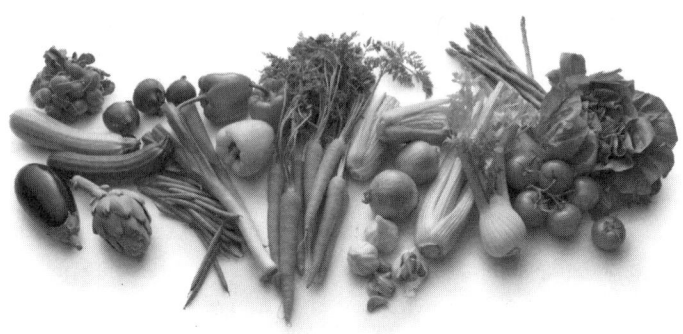

Sample Family Goal Contract

We the _____ family will work toward
_____ over the next 1 or 2 weeks.
When we have successfully made this a habit, we will reward ourselves with
_____.

Signed: _____
Date: _____

Keep track here:

Sunday	Monday	Tuesday	Wednesday	Thursday	Friday	Saturday

Take the Family Lifestyle Quiz

The Family Lifestyle Quiz will help you find changes you can make in your family environment. Answer "yes," "no," or "sometimes" to the following questions:

Do you and your family:	Yes	No	Sometimes
1. Have regularly scheduled mealtimes when you are home?			
2. Eat meals together at least once a day?			
3. Eat planned snacks (instead of just grabbing whatever is around when hungry)?			
4. Give portions sized to each person's needs?			
5. Plan and prepare meals together once a day?			
6. Eat three meals every day?			
7. Try to make mealtimes pleasant?			
8. Avoid making everyone eat everything on their plate before leaving the table?			
9. Make meals last more than 15 minutes?			
10. Eat only in designated areas of the house?			
11. Avoid using food to punish or reward?			
12. Enjoy physical activities together once or twice a week?			

Scoring the Quiz

Give yourself two points for every "yes" answer. Score one point for every "sometimes" answer. Give zero points for every "no" answer.

If you scored 20 to 24 points, your family is doing a great job in these areas! Read the next section for ways to make your skills stronger.

A score of 13 to 19 is good. But review the questions you answered "no" or "sometimes," and see what changes you can make. The next section provides helpful information on how to incorporate some of these changes in your home.

If your score is 12 points or fewer, following the suggestions in the next section can really help your child and your entire family.

Prepare Healthier Foods

Healthy eating needs to be a family affair. If you give special foods only to your overweight child, this can make him or her feel angry or ashamed.

All family members should eat healthy foods (see Box 4). Children are more likely to eat healthfully if they see you eating well—and your entire family will benefit from a healthier lifestyle.

 BOX 4   Six Keys to Healthy Eating

1. Make half your grains whole grains. Whole-wheat breads, oatmeal, brown rice, and low-fat popcorn are great options.

2. Make half your plate fruits and vegetables. Focus on whole fruits, vary your veggies, and include a variety of colors—like dark green, purple, red, and orange. Eat fresh, frozen, canned, or dried produce at meals and snacks.

3. Get calcium-rich foods. To build strong bones, include low-fat and fat-free milk products several times a day.

4. Go lean with protein. Eat lean or low-fat meat, chicken, turkey, and fish. Add dry beans and peas to salads, main dishes, and soups.

5. Change your oil. Use liquid oils for cooking—corn, peanut, safflower, soybean, canola, and olive oil are good choices.

6. Drink and eat less sodium, saturated fat, and added sugars. Choose foods and beverages that do not have sugar as one of the first ingredients.

Adapted from MyPlate, (www.choosemyplate.gov).

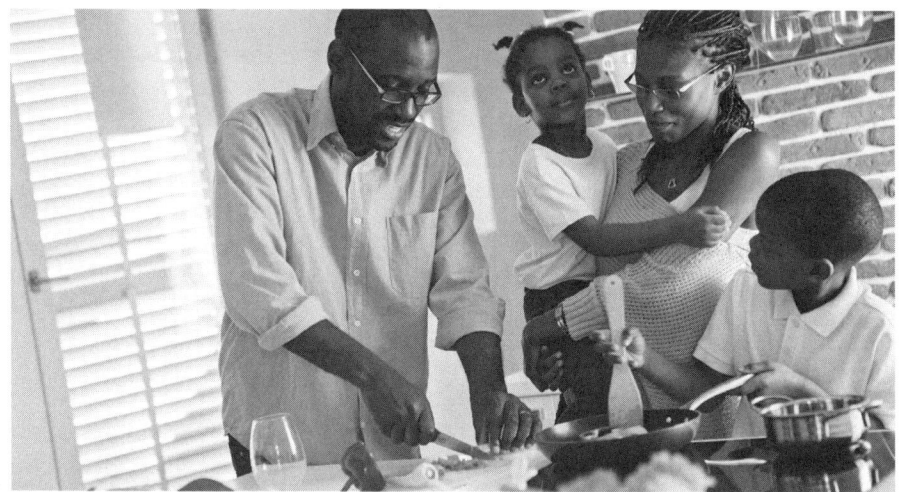

Plan and Prepare Meals Together

Involve your child in menu planning and meal preparation. This teaches your child about nutrition, which will help him or her to make his or her own food choices in the future. Additionally, children are more likely to eat, or at least try, foods that they help prepare.

A few tips for planning and preparing meals with your children include:

- Save your family's favorite menus and use them over and over again, making changes as needed.

- Be ready for your child to make a mistake or two, and let your child know that making mistakes is okay. Let your child try the recipe again sometime.

- Respect your child's tastes. For instance, many children don't like spicy food.

- Be aware that children may need to try new foods several times before they decide whether they really like them. As children grow up, they usually will eat more kinds of food.

Schedule Regular Mealtimes

Try to arrange your family's schedule so that meals can be served at predictable times. Without scheduled mealtimes, children tend to snack more on foods that are most convenient, which may be foods higher in calories, sugar, and fat. If regular family meals are not scheduled or are often missed, children may also overeat during the other meals of the day.

If your family can't always have an evening meal at the same time each day, that's okay. Make sure that each day your children are aware of the time it will be served, and if your evening meal is going to be a little late, plan for a slightly larger afternoon snack that day so your child does not get too hungry before the meal.

See Box 5 for tips on making family mealtime easier to plan.

 BOX 5 **Ways to Get Your Family Together at the Table**

Have breakfast together. Set the table the night before.

Pick at least one night a week to be family meal night. Keep a family calendar so everyone knows when it will be.

Plan ahead. Planned menus take some of the stress out of mealtimes.

Prepare foods ahead of time. Make casseroles, burritos, lasagna, meatloaf, or pasta ahead of time. Then reheat at mealtime.

Double your recipes. Freeze half to use at another time.

Use quick cooking methods. A microwave oven or pressure cooker can help. Prepare a crock pot in the morning and you will have a meal ready for dinnertime.

When you do sit down to eat together, try to make the meals last at least 15 minutes by eating more slowly (see Box 6). To feel satisfied at meals, you need to do a certain amount of tasting, chewing, and swallowing. When you eat quickly, you may need more food to feel satisfied. By eating more slowly, you can be satisfied with less food.

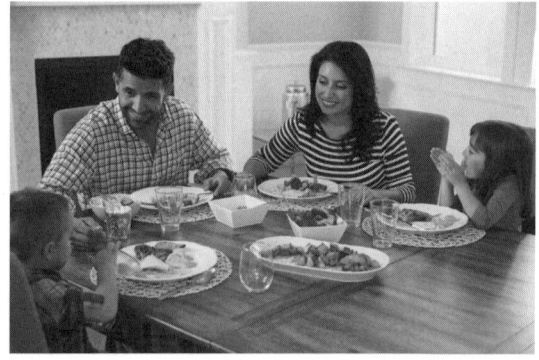

When your brain gets the message that your body is getting food, feelings of hunger will stop. This takes about 20 minutes. Fast eaters can eat a lot of food in that time.

BOX 6 Tips to Help Fast Eaters Slow Down

Put the spoon or fork down between bites.

Put finger foods (like sandwiches) down on the plate between bites.

Swallow what is in your mouth before you take another bite.

Take time for talking, resting, or taking a drink.

Take a sip of water between bites.

Stop eating for a minute once or twice during the meal. This will help break your eating rhythm. It also helps you to keep pace with slower eaters at the table.

If you want a second helping, wait five minutes. The desire may go away.

Make any second helpings half the size of the first.

Eat the meal in courses. Begin with the lowest calorie foods, such as fruits, vegetables, soups, and salads. This will help stop strong feelings of hunger. End the meal with higher calorie foods, such as breads, pastas, and meats.

Turn off distractions such as the TV and radio, and put away cell phones and tablets. Let voicemail pick up the telephone calls.

Encourage family sharing at mealtimes. After the meal starts, ask each person to talk about the best thing that happened to him or her that day.

Make Mealtime Pleasant

Mealtime should be a time when families get together and share with one another in a positive way. But, too often, mealtime can turn into scenes and arguments. Try setting rules against fighting or complaining at the table.

You may need to set aside a special time each week for the family to discuss problems. When mealtimes are stressful, children will eat fast so they can leave the table as soon as possible. They then begin to link eating with stress.

Avoid the Clean Plate Club

Some children believe that they need to finish their food to please their parents or to avoid punishment. For these kids, eating may become a performance issue instead of a way to be healthy and enjoy themselves.

Avoid being members of the "clean plate club." Help your children learn that they don't have to eat every bite of food that is placed in front of them. Instead, they should learn to eat until they feel satisfied.

Look back to the hunger scale on page 8 to help your child learn when to stop eating. You may also try letting your child make his or her own plate based on feelings of hunger.

Don't Use Food to Punish or Reward

When you need to discipline your child, do not do it with food. If you cut out food to punish a child, this can make your child feel anxious. Your child may worry that he or she will not get enough food or go hungry. As a result, your child may often overeat at meals or try to eat snacks whenever there is a chance.

Similarly, do not use food as a reward. Children may come to expect more dessert when they try new foods or clean their plates. Also, when children are rewarded with sweets or snack food, they may decide that these foods are better or more valuable than healthier foods. This belief is especially hard to break and may continue throughout your child's life. Instead, try some food-free rewards such as:

- Having a friend stay overnight

- Time alone with mom or dad

- A new book

- A trip to the movies

- A day at the pool, roller rink, or bowling alley

Enjoy Physical Activities Together

Physical activity helps to control weight. It has other benefits too.

 BOX 7 **Benefits of Physical Activity**

Helps control appetite

Lowers stress

Builds strength

Reduces risk of diseases such as diabetes and heart disease

Improves health

Increases social contact

Burns calories

Helps you deal with emotions and feelings

May improve academic performance

Centers for Disease Control and Prevention

Try to involve the whole family in physical activity. Your child is more likely to be active if you are active.

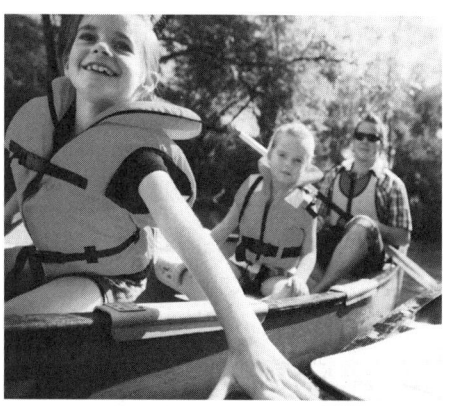

Choose some of your family's favorite activities, and come up with a few new ones (see Box 8, page 20). Then decide how many times each week you can add them to your activity schedule. Work up to 60 minutes of physical activity per day, 5 to 7 days a week.

BOX 8 **Family Activity Ideas**

Archery	Freeze tag	Playing at the park
Badminton	Frisbee	Rollerblading
Batting practice	Golf lessons	Running
Basketball	Hacky sack	Running through the sprinkler
Biking	Hiking	
Bowling	Hockey	Sledding
Building a sandcastle or snowman	Hopscotch	Soccer
	Ice skating	Softball
Canoeing	Jump rope	Snowshoeing
Catch	Kayaking	Swimming
Catching butterflies or frogs	Kickball	T-ball
Croquet	Kite flying	Tennis
Dancing	Miniature golf	Track and field sports
Fishing	Paddle boating	Walking
Football	Ping pong	Water slide

Before you begin family activities or encourage your child to become more active, keep the following points in mind:

- Overweight children may not feel comfortable in organized and competitive games. Choose activities where winning or performing well don't matter (like biking or walking the dog).

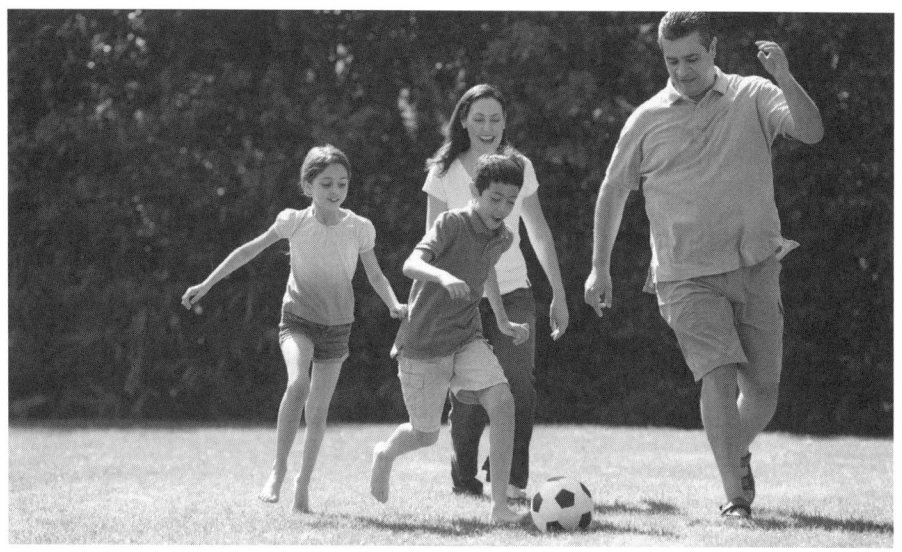

- More activity won't just happen. You need to help your child plan for it. Plan a family walk right after dinner. Arrange a family activity on weekends.

- Physical activity can be increased small ways. When you go to the store, park farther away and walk. Take the stairs instead of the elevator. Or have your child push the shopping cart if he or she is able. Even daily chores can burn calories. (See Box 9, page 22, for some ideas.)

- Be sure that activities are safe and that the right gear is used. For example, children should ride on bike paths if available and wear bike helmets. Also, make sure your child has a water bottle, especially in hot weather.

- Choose fun activities. When children have fun while exercising, they are more likely to continue enjoying it for the rest of their lives.

- Let your child try lots of activities. Offer choices like baseball, basketball, tennis, track and field, or soccer. Then let him or her choose what he or she likes to do best.

- Teach moderation in exercise. Exercise should be fun and healthy. It should not be an obsession. It should not cause injuries.

- Schedule fitness into family vacations. Whether it's hiking or swimming, make sure your vacation includes some daily activity.

BOX 9 Daily Activities That Can Burn Calories

Bagging leaves	Pushing a shopping cart
Playing with the dog	Pushing a stroller with a baby in it
Carrying and stacking wood	Raking leaves and jumping in them
Cleaning your room or the game room	Shoveling snow
Cleaning windows	Vacuuming
Mopping the floor	Walking the dog
Dusting	Walking fast
Gardening and weeding	Washing the car with mom or dad
Mowing the lawn	Washing dishes

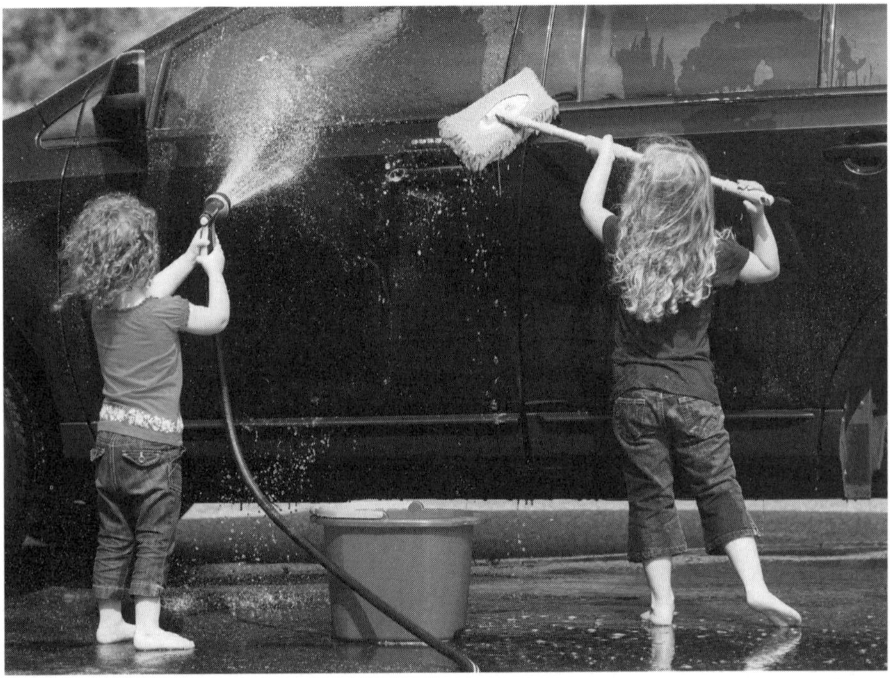

PORTIONS AND SNACKS

Portion sizes for meals and snacks are important to keep in mind. If children are given larger portion sizes, they tend to eat more.

Match Portions to Your Child's Needs

Younger children need smaller portions of food than adults, while older children may need portions that are closer to an adult serving. Table 1 offers some examples of appropriate portion sizes for different foods, and ways to measure without weighing or using measuring cups. Use this guide to help track recommended daily amounts from each food group, discussed in the next chapter.

Table 1: Average Portion Guide

Food	Average Portion Size	Looks Like the Size of . . .
Milk, yogurt	1 cup	An adult fist
Hard cheese	1 ounce	Four dice
Meat, poultry, fish	2 to 3 ounces (cooked)	A deck of cards
Peanut butter	2 tablespoons	A ping pong ball
Fresh fruit	1 piece	A baseball or tennis ball
Canned fruit	½ cup	Half a baseball
Pasta or rice	½ cup	A tennis ball or ice cream scoop
Salad greens	1 cup	Amount an adult could hold in two cupped hands
Baked potato	1 small	An adult fist or light bulb

Help your child become more aware of sensible portion sizes. Try using smaller cups, bowls, and plates for your child, which can help portions look bigger. Your children may be nervous that the allotted portion sizes will not fill them up, so be sure to let them know that once they are finished, they will have a chance for seconds (keeping in mind the rule that seconds should be half the size of the original portion). When serving snacks, always portion out an appropriate amount rather than eating directly from a package or large serving container.

Plan for Snacks

Snacking is okay. Planned snacks at specific times of the day can be part of a healthy diet and will not spoil your child's appetite at mealtimes—in fact, snacks may keep your child from getting too hungry between meals and then overeating. But too much snacking can lead to extra calories, and so you can run into problems with snacking if you are unprepared. Snack smart by keeping the following points in mind:

- Most children need just two or maybe three snacks per day.

- Offer snacks at least 1 hour before mealtime, that way your child will be hungry at meals.

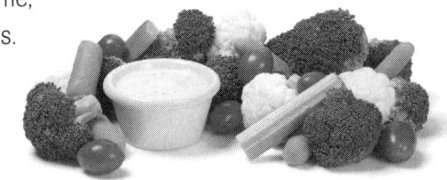

- It's good to be hungry at mealtimes. It will encourage your child to try new foods.

- If your child is not hungry at meals, skip the snacks, serve them earlier, or make them smaller.

- Snacks are not meals. A half sandwich, a piece of fruit, or a small bowl of cereal is probably enough food.

- Children shouldn't snack in front of the TV or computer or while playing video games. These activities make it difficult to pay attention to feelings of fullness.

- Snacks should be eaten only in selected areas such as the kitchen or dining room.

- Make sure to have the right snack foods on hand. You and your child can develop a list of snacks together. When your child needs a snack, he or she can choose something from that list.

Unplanned snacks can be a problem because children get hungry and eat any food that grabs their attention. These foods are often "convenience foods" that are high in fat and/or sugar (for example, crackers, potato chips, ice cream bars, candy bars, and gummy fruit snacks). Don't purchase these items or have them in your house.

Try the following healthier snack ideas:

- Raw vegetables with low-fat dip or low-calorie salad dressing

- Fresh fruit

- Canned fruit (in its own juice, not in syrup)

- Unsweetened applesauce

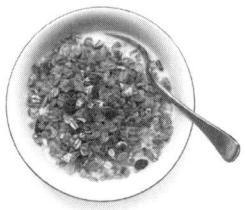

- Dry cereal with low-fat milk

- Reduced-fat cheese with low-fat crackers

- Unbuttered or light microwave popcorn (Do not give to children younger than 5 years.)

- Pretzels or whole grain crackers with cheese dip

- Low-fat yogurt, plain yogurt mixed with fruit, or a mix of nonfat plain and flavored yogurts

- Graham crackers with low-fat hot chocolate

- Half of a sandwich made with meat, light mayonnaise, mustard, tomato, and lettuce

- Animal crackers

- Gingersnaps or vanilla wafers

- English muffin pizza (half a muffin topped with tomato sauce and low-fat cheese)

- One frozen waffle with fresh fruit

- A small whole wheat bagel (or half a bagel) spread lightly with low-fat margarine or natural peanut butter and low-sugar jelly

- Instant noodle or vegetable soup

- A small baked potato with low-fat sour cream or low-fat margarine

- A tossed salad with low-fat dressing

- Pudding made with low-fat milk

- A 100%-fruit-juice popsicle

- String cheese made from low-fat mozzarella

- A soft pretzel with mustard

- A small whole wheat tortilla rolled up with meat, low-fat mayonnaise, lettuce, and tomato

Eat Only in Designated Areas of the House

Your family should only eat meals and snacks in the kitchen or the dining room. This will help your family to eat less often because it will prevent them from mindlessly eating in front of the TV or computer, and it will make them more aware of how often they are eating.

Your family should also sit down whenever they eat. If you eat standing up, you pay less attention to portion size. When you sit down and focus on eating, you are more aware of what you are eating, which may help your child eat smaller amounts.

Store Food Out of Sight

Keep food out of sight until mealtime or snack time. The sight of food makes many children (and adults) want to eat.

Remove easy-to-eat foods from the kitchen counter. For example, if you have a cookie jar, move it to a hard-to-reach spot in the pantry or cupboard. For foods like crackers or cereal, where it may be tempting to eat these straight from a bag or box, portion these into snack-size bags to make it easier to control the amount eaten at one time.

Keep healthy foods where they will be easy to access. Great foods to keep on hand are fresh fruit, baby carrots, single-size fruit cups, and low-fat yogurt.

NUTRITIONAL NEEDS OF GROWING CHILDREN

Children grow quickly. As your child grows, he or she needs the right amount of calories, protein, vitamins, and minerals.

Instead of cutting foods and calories out of your child's eating plan, help him or her learn how to replace higher-calorie, less nutritious foods with a variety of healthy lower-calorie foods. Your child should eat foods from all the different food groups each day:

- Grains

- Vegetables

- Fruits

- Milk

- Protein Foods

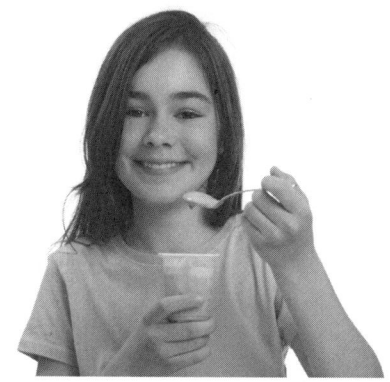

The 2015-2020 Dietary Guidelines for Americans and Choose MyPlate are good sources of information on the types and amounts of food that are right for different calorie levels, based on age, sex, and activity level. To learn more about the food groups and how to build healthier eating habits, visit the MyPlate website at www.ChooseMyPlate.gov.

Table 2 (page 28) suggests a range of recommended calories for boys and girls ages 4 to 12. The amount your child needs will vary based on level of activity. The lower end of the range is for children who get very little physical activity, while the higher end of the range is for very active children. An RDN can help you identify the right calorie level for your child.

Table 2: Daily Calorie Levels for Children Ages 4-12

Age	Boys	Girls
4	1,200-1,600	1,200-1,400
5	1,200-1,600	1,200-1,600
6	1,400-1,800	1,200-1,600
7	1,400-1,800	1,200-1,800
8	1,400-2,000	1,400-1,800
9	1,600-2,000	1,400-1,800
10	1,600-2,200	1,400-2,000
11	1,800-2,200	1,600-2,000
12	1,800-2,400	1,600-2,200

2015-2020 Dietary Guidelines for Americans

Once you know the daily calorie goal for your child, you can use Table 3 to find the right amounts of food per food group at each calorie level. The daily amounts from each food group are recommended to help meet your child's energy and nutrient needs.

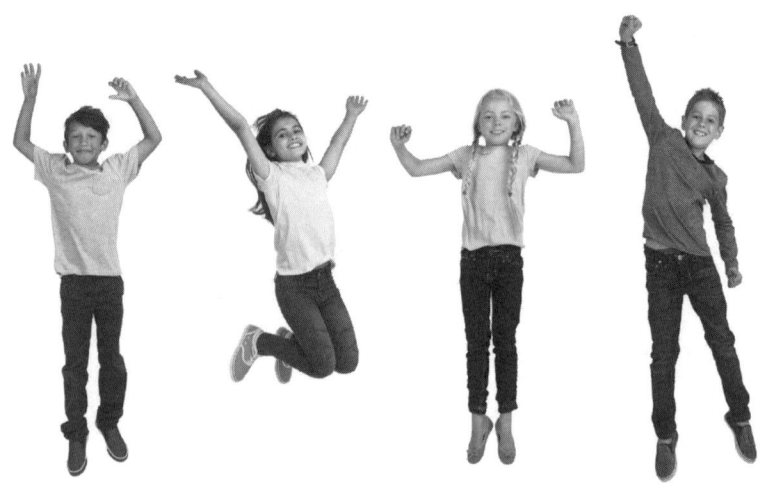

Table 3: Recommended Daily Amounts from Each Food Group

Calories per Day	Grains[a]	Vegetables[b]	Fruits[b]	Dairy[c]	Protein Foods[d]	Limits on Extras (Added Fats & Sweets)[e]
1,200	4 ounces	1½ cups	1 cup	2½ cups	3 ounces	100 calories
1,400	5 ounces	1½ cups	1½ cups	2½ cups	4 ounces	110 calories
1,600	5 ounces	2 cups	1½ cups	3 cups	5 ounces	130 calories
1,800	6 ounces	2½ cups	1½ cups	3 cups	5 ounces	170 calories
2,000	6 ounces	2½ cups	2 cups	3 cups	5½ ounces	270 calories
2,200	7 ounces	3 cups	2 cups	3 cups	6 ounces	280 calories
2,400	8 ounces	3 cups	2 cups	3 cups	6½ ounces	350 calories

[a] 1 ounce of grains is equal to: ½ cup of cooked rice, pasta, or cereal; 1 ounce of dry pasta or rice; 1 medium (1 ounce) slice of bread; 1 ounce of ready-to-eat cereal (about 1 cup of flaked cereal).

[b] 1 cup of fruits or vegetables is equal to 1 cup of raw or cooked vegetable or fruit; 1 cup of vegetable or fruit juice; 2 cups of leafy salad greens, ½ cup of dried fruit or vegetable.

[c] 1 cup of dairy is equal to 1 cup of low-fat or fat-free milk, yogurt, or fortified soymilk; 1½ ounces of natural cheese such as cheddar or Swiss cheese; 2 ounces of processed cheese such as American.

[d] 1 ounce of protein foods is equal to 1 ounce of lean meat, poultry, or seafood; 1 egg; ¼ cup of cooked beans or tofu; 1 tablespoon of peanut or nut butter; ½ ounce of nuts or seeds.

[e] Calories for extras can only be included if all foods selected from each food group are lean or low-fat and prepared without added fats, sugars, or refined starches.

2015-2020 Dietary Guidelines for Americans

Eat Less Fat and Less *Trans* Fat

Our bodies need a certain amount of fat to stay healthy. For children, the body uses fat to:

- Grow

- Store energy

- Heal wounds

- Protect organs such as the heart, liver, and kidneys

- Absorb certain vitamins (vitamins A, D, E, and K)

However, most children get more than enough fat from the foods they eat. Too much fat can provide excess calories, and diets that are high in fat, especially saturated fat and *trans* fat, are linked to high blood cholesterol, obesity, and diabetes.

Eating less fat is a good way to cut calories without cutting out nutrients or going hungry. To get less fat, choose nonfat or low-fat dairy products, lean meats and poultry, and low-fat or fat-free salad dressings and margarine. Table 4 lists some common foods that are high in fat and suggests lower-fat choices that are also lower in calories.

Table 4: Fat Facts

Food Group	Higher-Fat Foods	Lower-Fat Choices
Oils	Butter and margarine	Use light cream cheese or low-calorie tub margarine without *trans* fats
	Sour cream	Reduced-fat sour cream
	Mayonnaise	Low-fat mayonnaise
	Salad dressings	Reduced-fat dressings
	Oil for cooking or frying	Broth, juice, nonstick spray
	Beef or pork fat, lard	Olive, canola, soybean, or safflower oil

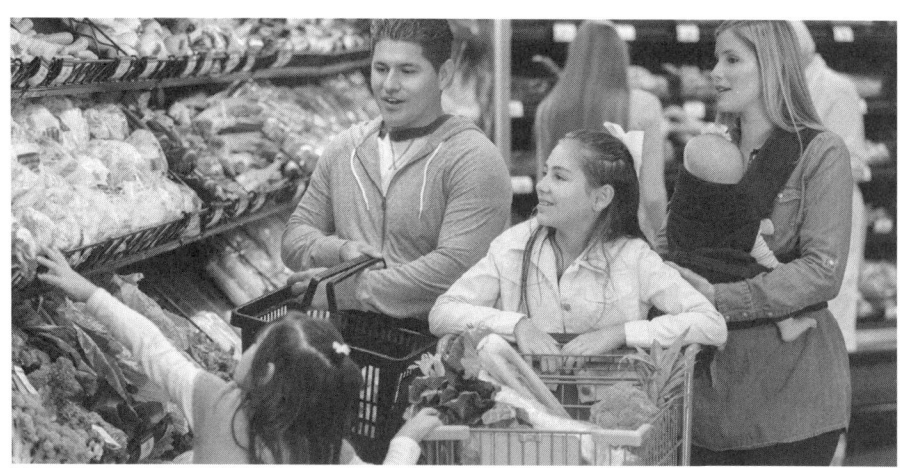

Food Group	Higher-Fat Foods	Lower-Fat Choices
Protein Foods	Bacon	Canadian bacon, turkey or chicken bacon
	Ground beef	95% lean beef, ground turkey or chicken breast
	Prime cuts of beef	"Choice" or " select" grades of beef (cut off any fat that you see)
	Poultry with skin	Poultry with skin removed before eating
	Fried fish	Baked or broiled fish
	Tuna in oil	Tuna packed in water
Milk	Whole or 2% milk	Nonfat (skim) or 1% milk
	Yogurt	Nonfat or low-fat yogurt
	Cheese	Cheese with 2 to 6 grams of fat per ounce
	Cottage cheese, ricotta cheese	Low-fat cottage cheese, low-fat ricotta
	Cream	Evaporated skim milk

Food Group	Higher-Fat Foods	Lower-Fat Choices
Snacks and Sweets	Cakes	Angel food cake, unfrosted cakes, baked apples, poached pears, fig bars
	Cookies	Animal crackers, vanilla wafers, gingersnaps, graham crackers, fig bars (look for choices made without *trans* fat)
	Pudding	Pudding made with nonfat (skim) milk
	Candy bars	15 jelly beans, a lollypop, licorice, or two hard candies
	Ice cream	Low-fat ice cream or frozen yogurt, popsicles, or light fudgesicles
	Potato chips	Baked potato chips, pretzels, low-fat crackers
	Buttered popcorn	Light microwave popcorn or air-popped popcorn
	Croissant	Small bagel or pita bread

All types of fat contain the same amount of calories, but some types are healthier than others. When cutting back on fat, focus especially on cutting back on saturated fat and *trans* fat. These types of fat can raise the level of cholesterol in the blood, which may increase the risk of heart disease.

Saturated fat is found in animal foods (the fat inside and around meats and poultry) and in dairy foods like whole milk, cheese, and butter. It is also found in palm and coconut oils. Lean meats and lower-fat dairy foods have less saturated fat. Saturated fat is usually solid at room temperature and is sometimes referred to as a "solid fat."

Trans fats may occur naturally, in small amounts, in some animal products, such as meat, whole milk, and milk products. However most *trans* fats are formed when liquid vegetable oils go through a process that changes them from liquid to solid. This is called "hydrogenation." To find out if a food has *trans* fat, look for the words "partially hydrogenated" on the ingredient list. If you see these words, there is some *trans* fat in the product. Many food companies are removing *trans* fat from processed foods, but they may often still contain saturated fat.

The amounts of saturated and *trans* fats in one serving of food are listed on the food's Nutrition Facts label. Compare products and choose foods that are low in these fats. Try to replace saturated fats with unsaturated fats, such as those found in oils, soft margarine, nuts, and seeds, whenever possible. Unsaturated fats are better for your heart and are usually liquid at room temperature. For example, canola oil is an excellent oil to use in cooking and baking, and olive oil is good for stir-frying and salad dressings.

Nutrition Facts

8 servings per container
Serving size 2/3 cup (55g)

Amount per serving
Calories 230

	% Daily Value*
Total Fat 8g	**10%**
Saturated Fat 1g	**5%**
Trans Fat 0g	
Cholesterol 0mg	**0%**
Sodium 160mg	**7%**
Total Carbohydrate 37g	**13%**
Dietary Fiber 4g	**14%**
Total Sugars 12g	
Includes 10g Added Sugars	**20%**
Protein 3g	
Vitamin D 2mcg	10%
Calcium 260mg	20%
Iron 8mg	45%
Potassium 235mg	6%

* The % Daily Value (DV) tells you how much a nutrient in a serving of food contributes to a daily diet. 2,000 calories a day is used for general nutrition advice.

Eat Less Sugar and Drink Fewer Sugary Beverages

If your child eats a variety of foods, an occasional sweet can be included in your child's diet. But some children consume too many sweet foods and beverages, and this can lead to excess calories and weight gain. Also, if a child eats too many sweets, he or she can miss out on foods rich in vitamins, minerals, fiber, and protein. Foods containing lots of sugar are usually high in calories and fat, and they are often low in nutrients.

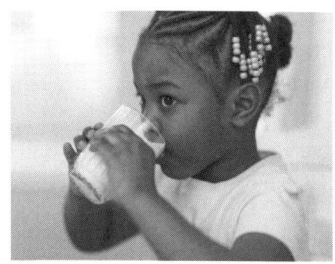

Added sugar should make up less than 10% of daily calories for both children and adults. For example, a child who consumes 1,600 calories per day should have no more than 40 grams of added sugars per day in order to keep added sugar at less than 10% of his or her daily calories. To calculate, multiply your child's recommended calories by 10%, then divide this by 4 to find out the daily grams of added sugars, or see Table 5 (page 34). Naturally occurring sugars such as those in fruit or milk products (plain milk or yogurt) are not added sugars and are not included in this recommended limit.

Table 5: Daily Limits for Added Sugars

Calories	Added Sugars (grams) at Less than 10% of Daily Calories:
1,200	30
1,400	35
1,600	40
1,800	45
2,000	50
2,200	55
2,400	60

To find out whether a food contains added sugar, first check the ingredients listed on the label. They are listed in order from largest to smallest amount. If sugar is one of the first three or four ingredients, the food is probably high in sugar. Box 10 gives examples of other names for added sugars. Next, look at the grams of added sugar listed on the Nutrition Facts label (required on labels by 2018) to help judge how this food will contribute to daily added sugar intake.

You probably know that foods such as soda, candy, sweetened fruit juice or canned fruit, fruit drinks, and desserts can contain a lot of sugar. To help reduce added sugars, instead choose drinks like water, 100% juice, or reduced-sugar or sugar-free juice drinks. Other sweetened foods can be included, but just be aware of your child's daily limits and the amount of sugar in the portion your child eats or drinks.

 BOX 10   Examples of Added Sugars

Labels for sweetened foods don't always list "sugar" as an ingredient. Other types of added sugar that you may see on an ingredient list include fructose, corn sweetener, corn syrup, high fructose corn syrup, fruit juice concentrate, sucrose, honey, sugar, invert sugar, maple syrup, sorghum, brown sugar, molasses, lactose, maltose, malt syrup, dextrose, or glucose.

Eat More Whole Grains and Fiber

Wheat, rice, oats, and barley are grains. There are two main types of grain products: whole grain and refined. Whole grains contain all the parts of the grain (the whole grain). Refined grains have been milled, which removes the bran and germ parts of the grain—the parts of the grain that contain vitamins, iron, and fiber.

Grain-based foods made from refined flour, including most noodles, many crackers, white bread, flour tortillas, pita bread, white rice, and many breakfast cereals, still provide important nutrients. In these foods, nutrients such as B vitamins and iron, and other nutrients that are lost when flour is refined, are added. However, the fiber that is lost is not added back.

Fiber helps to prevent heart disease and some types of cancer and can also help control diabetes. It helps prevent constipation and makes foods more filling to eat.

The fiber recommendation for children age 4 to 8 years old is 25 grams per day. For 9 to 13 year old girls, 26 grams of fiber per day is recommended, while boys age 9 to13 need 31 grams of fiber each day. Whole grains, along with whole fruits and vegetables, beans, and legumes, help us reach the recommended daily amounts of fiber. A good rule of thumb is that at least half of the grain foods that your child eats should be whole grain foods. Look for products that have whole wheat or whole grain as the first ingredient on the food label.

Good whole grain choices are:

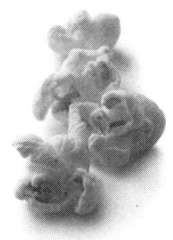

- Whole grain breads and cereals

- Brown rice and wild rice

- Other whole grains like quinoa, barley, bulgur, and millet

- Whole grain crackers

- Popcorn

- Oatmeal

Many ready-to-eat breakfast cereals are made with whole grains. These cereals often look the same as products made without whole grain. Check the Nutrition Facts label to see if they have more fiber. However, some cereals made with whole grains are high in sugar. To get less sugar and more fiber, try mixing a high-fiber cereal with a little bit of a sweet one.

SAMPLE MENUS

Menu planning makes mealtimes run more smoothly. When you decide in advance what you are going to serve, then no one has to figure out what they "feel like" eating. Also, you can make healthier meals when you plan ahead.

The six sample menu plans in this booklet are for children of different age groups. These menus are based on recommended amounts from each food group for different calories levels (Table 3, page 29). An RDN can help you create a meal plan that is right for your child.

When you start out, plan just a few breakfasts and lunches. It's even okay for your breakfasts and lunches to be the same every day at first—you can always add more choices later.

Focus on planning several dinner menus. Try starting with 10 healthy meals for dinners, and rotate these. You can then add more options as you come up with new ideas for healthy meals that your family might enjoy.

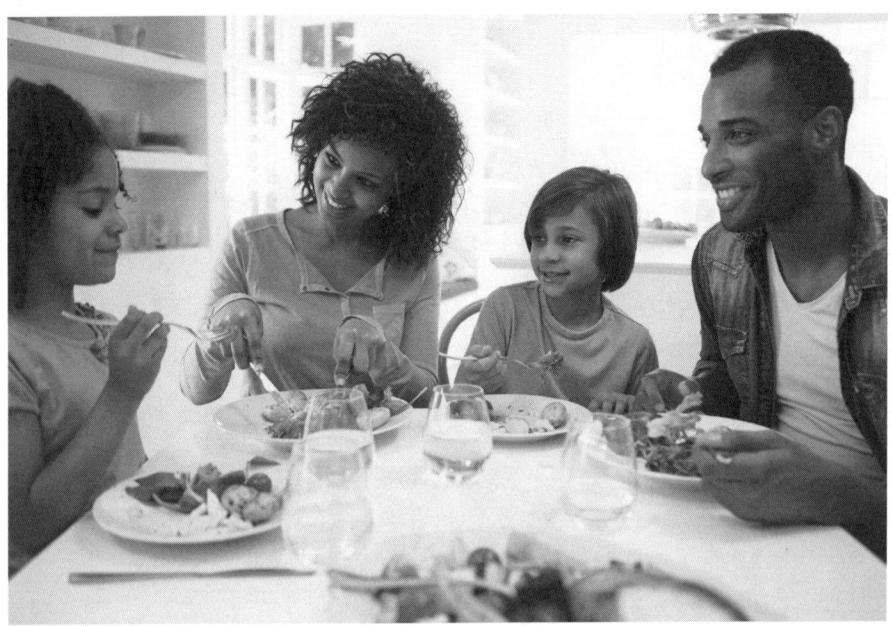

Sample Menu 1: For Kids Ages 4 to 6 Years

Breakfast

½ banana

1 cup low-fat milk

1 cup toasted oat cereal made with whole grains

Lunch

¼ apple

1 cup low-fat milk

1 or 2 slices whole grain bread

2 ounces turkey

6 or 7 baby carrots

Dinner

¼ cup strawberries

½ cup green beans

½ cup pasta

2 ounces meatballs

½ cup tomato sauce

Water

Snacks

½ cup (4 ounces) low-fat yogurt

5 to 7 vanilla wafers

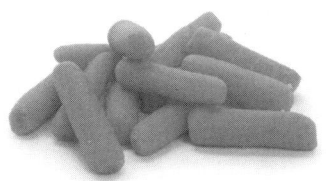

Sample Menu 2: For Kids Ages 4 to 6 Years

Breakfast

½ cup orange juice

2 slices whole wheat toast

1 to 2 tablespoons peanut butter

Lunch

1 wheat tortilla

1 ounce grilled chicken with taco seasoning

1 ounce reduced-fat cheese, shredded

Shredded lettuce, diced tomato

15 grapes

Water

Dinner

½ cup fried rice

1 to 2 ounces beef stir-fried with ½ cup broccoli and plum sauce

1 cup nonfat chocolate milk

Snacks

1 ounce reduced-fat cheese with whole grain crackers

1 kiwi fruit

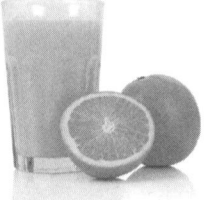
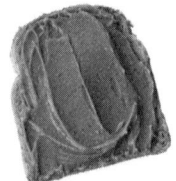

Sample Menu 3: For Kids Ages 7 to 9 Years

Breakfast

½ cup blueberries

2 pancakes

2 teaspoons low-calorie syrup

½ cup low-fat milk

Lunch

1 whole wheat bun

½ cup barbecued shredded pork

½ cup oven-baked fries

¼ cup whole kernel corn

4 apple slices

½ cup low-fat milk

Dinner

⅓ cup brown rice

Kabob made with 2 ounces grilled chicken and ½ cup potato, green pepper, and tomato

½ cup unsweetened pineapple

Water

Snacks

1 ounce low-fat string cheese

½ cup low-fat milk and 1 graham cracker

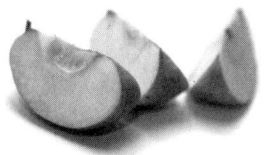

Sample Menu 4: For Kids Ages 7 to 9 Years

Breakfast

½ grapefruit

½ cup cooked oatmeal

½ cup low-fat milk

Lunch

1 wheat pita pocket

2 ounces turkey

Lettuce, tomato

Mustard or light mayonnaise

1 cup low-fat milk

1 orange

Dinner

1 cup pasta

2 ounces cheese sauce

½ cup broccoli

1 watermelon slice

Water

Snacks

Celery sticks with 1 tablespoon peanut butter

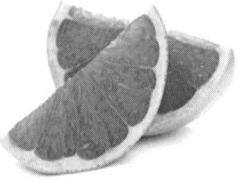 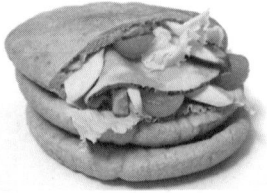 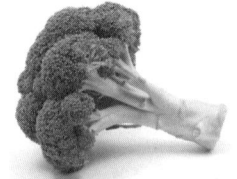

Sample Menu 5: For Kids Ages 10 to 12 Years

Breakfast

12 grapes

1 whole wheat bagel

2 tablespoons peanut butter

1 cup nonfat (skim) milk

Lunch

1 apple

1 to 2 whole wheat hot dog bun(s)

1 to 2 low-fat or nonfat hot dogs or turkey dogs

Ketchup, mustard, and relish

½ cup oven-baked fries

1 cup non-fat (skim) milk

Dinner

½ cup berries

1 burrito (tortilla, 2 ounces shredded chicken, 1 ounce reduced-fat cheese,
¼ cup low-fat refried beans, salsa)

½ cup Spanish rice

Small tossed salad with 1 to 2 ounces low-fat dressing

Water

Snacks

½ cup (4 ounces) low-fat yogurt

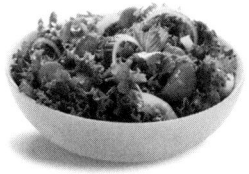

Sample Menu 6: For Kids Ages 10 to 12 Years

Breakfast

1 small banana

1 cup low-fat milk

1 to 2 cups ready-to-eat whole grain cereal

Lunch

1 pear

6-inch whole wheat bun

2 ounces roast turkey

1 ounce reduced-fat cheese

Lettuce, cucumber slices, tomato, green pepper, olives, mustard

1-ounce bag baked potato chips

Water

Dinner

1 or 2 Chinese pancakes

2 ounces moo shu chicken with onions and moo shu sauce

½ cup steamed brown rice

½ to 1 cup stir-fried vegetables

1 cup low-fat milk

Snacks

1 cup strawberries with 1 tablespoon low-fat whipped cream

SPECIAL SITUATIONS

There are times when children may be tempted by less healthful foods. You can help your child learn how to deal with such situations.

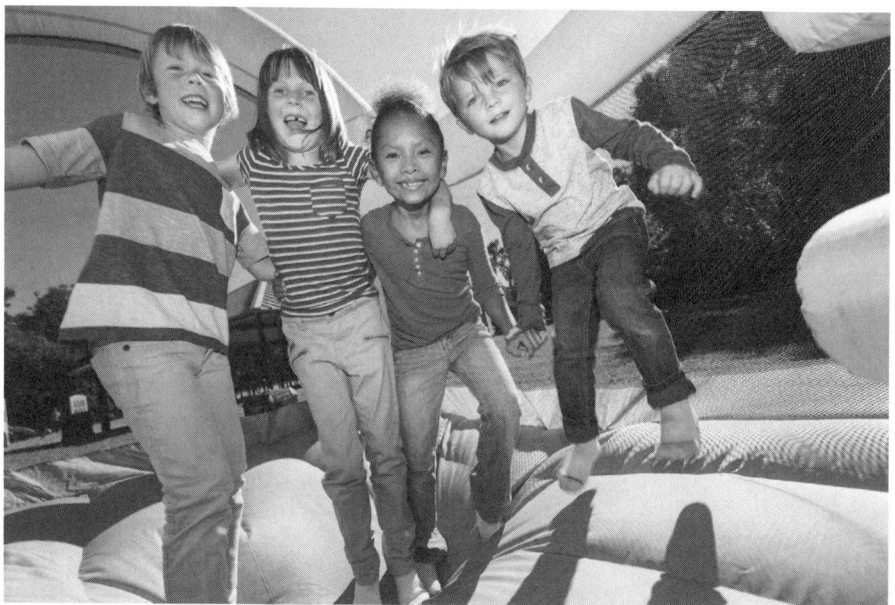

Parties and Holidays

Special events such as birthday parties are important to kids. Overweight children should be able to enjoy events even though high-calorie foods such as cake, candy, and ice cream may be served. If you are planning a kids party, make it an active one. For example, you can have the party at the roller rink, bowling alley, or playground.

Holidays can be a different challenge. Depending on the time of year or the holidays celebrated, there can be several "special" days in a row. Talk with your child about which days he or she would like to celebrate in the usual way, and think of new ways to celebrate the other days. You could go swimming or sledding, or you could walk around the zoo. Instead of baking cookies, make crafts and gifts. You can also try incorporating different foods into celebrations. In the winter, kids may enjoy fresh fruit just as much as cakes, cookies, and candies.

Time with Relatives

Relatives may offer special foods or treats to children, usually as a way to show affection. It's important for you to help your child learn how to deal directly with relatives who may seem to encourage eating large portions or too many treats.

Try role playing with your child so he or she can practice dealing with someone who frequently offers him or her food. Encourage your child to ask relatives and friends for help.

For example, your child may say, "Grandma, the kids at school tease me and call me names because of my weight. It's really hard in gym class when I don't do very well. I want to change. But I need your help to stop eating treats. Maybe we could go for a walk instead of having cookies and ice cream." It is likely that your relatives will want to support your child once they learn how he or she feels.

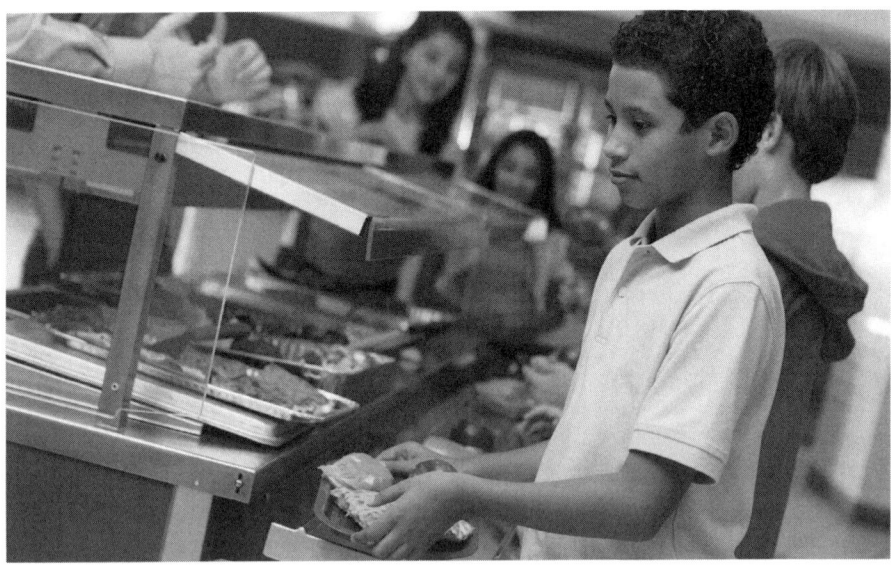

School Lunch

A school lunch program can be convenient, and it can also teach children about food, portions, and health.

Many schools try to have several healthy options as part of their school lunch program. If your child eats school lunches, check what is on the menu. You can talk with your child about which options he or she should choose, and it will help you to plan snacks that fit with the lunch choices. Remind your child that he or she does not need to eat everything on the plate.

Sometimes children really want to take lunch to school. To help make mornings go smoother, prepare lunches the night before. A week's worth of sandwiches can be made in advance and put in the freezer, and if you take one out each morning, it will thaw by noon. If you are packing leftovers and want to freshen things up, you can add some fruit or veggies as a snack, and your child can buy low-fat milk at school.

Even when bringing a healthy lunch from home, your child may be tempted to trade foods with other children or may ask to bring chips, cookies, or soda like some of his or her friends. It can help for your child to eat a decent-sized healthy breakfast so he or she isn't starving by lunchtime and it might be easier to turn down some of those foods. Another option is to pack small portions of a favorite food or treat at lunch. Sometimes just a few bites is enough to satisfy the desire for these foods.

Eating Out

When your family dines out, you and your children may find it to be more difficult to control calories and eat less fat. For instance, the foods that kids order most often are soft drinks and French fries. A regular soft drink contains about 120 calories—or about 30 grams of added sugar—and a small order of fries has 240 calories and about 11 grams of fat.

Many restaurants offer lower fat, lower calorie versions of regular items. They also have light or diet menus, and often serve low-fat milk.

Use the following tips to choose more healthful foods when eating out.

Breakfast

- Pancakes can be a good choice. It's fine to have about two tablespoons of syrup, but skip the butter.

- Order an English muffin or a bagel instead of a croissant, biscuit, or Danish pastry. Add only a small amount of jelly.

- Stick with Canadian bacon or ham instead of sausage or bacon.

- Watch out for oversized, high-calorie muffins and bagels. Some muffins and bagels have as many calories and as much fat as doughnuts.

- Choose low-fat or fat-free milk, a small orange juice, or water.

Lunch and Dinner

- Ask for reduced-calorie salad dressings.

- Hold the mayonnaise or special sauce, and skip the cheese on burgers and sandwiches. Use ketchup, mustard, or barbecue sauce instead.

- Stick with baked, broiled, or poached items.

- Avoid breaded and fried items such as fish sticks or chicken nuggets.

- Ask that sauces, dressings, gravy, butter, or sour cream be served on the side. Then, use just a little. Choose low-fat when available.

- Ask for substitutions. Many restaurants can serve a baked potato, raw vegetables, fruit, or a salad instead of fries or coleslaw.

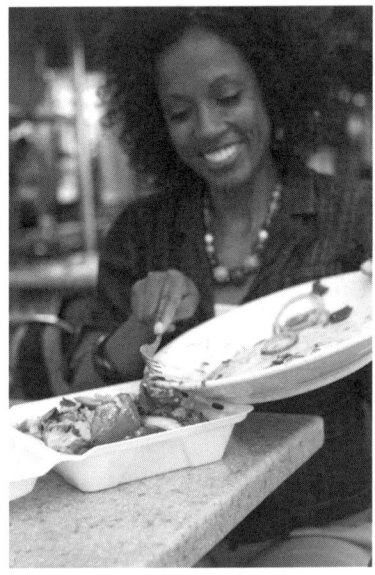

- Order à la carte (one item at a time) to get only what you want. Daily specials are often loaded with high-calorie items.

- Watch portion sizes. In many restaurants, portions are large enough for two children to share.

- If portions are large, ask for a take-out container. Put some of the food in the container before you start eating.

- Ask that bread, drinks, and chips be served with the meal, not before it. Hungry children may finish their drinks and fill up on bread, butter, and chips while they wait for their meals.

- Keep kids busy with crayons and paper while the food is being prepared, or have a tic-tac-toe contest with older children.

- Skip menu items described as buttery, in butter sauce, fried, pan-fried, crispy, creamed, in cream sauce, in gravy, with hollandaise, au gratin, in cheese sauce, or marinated in oil. These terms mean high-calorie, high-fat foods.

- Order thin-crust pizza with cheese and vegetables. Choose Canadian bacon instead of sausage or pepperoni.

- Ask about how foods are prepared. Feel free to request special orders.

- Order low-fat milk, fruit juice, or water instead of a soft drink or a milkshake.

Fast Food Best Bets

- Fruit or vegetable salad with low-fat dressing on the side

- Fresh fruit or applesauce

- Low-fat or fat-free milk instead of soda

- Grilled chicken sandwich without mayonnaise or with low-fat mayonnaise

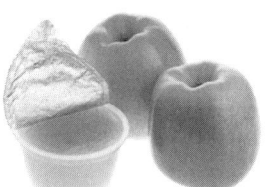

- Roast beef sandwich with barbecue sauce

- Submarine or deli sandwiches with lean meat or vegetables but without dressings or cheese (Ask for mustard or light mayonnaise instead. Skip meat salad sandwiches.)

- Chicken or steak soft tacos (Skip fried tortillas and the sour cream. Add mild salsa instead.)

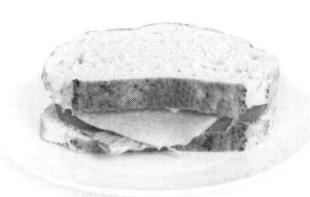

- Garden vegetable or Greek stuffed pitas (Go light on the cucumber sauce.)

- A small hamburger with ketchup, mustard, pickle, lettuce, tomato, and onion

- Broth-based soups, such as chicken noodle or minestrone

- Grilled veggie burgers (Skip the mayonnaise and cheese.)

- Baked potato (Go easy on the sour cream and margarine. Ask for light sour cream.)

- French dip sandwiches without the cheese

- A small serving (½ cup) of frozen low-fat yogurt or low-fat ice cream

- Baked beans, corn on the cob, mashed potatoes

- Chili, corn muffins, tossed salad, orange slices

- Split a small order of French fries

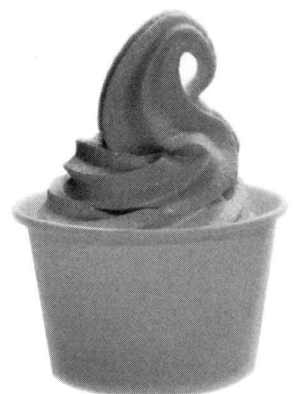

WEIGHT MANAGEMENT PROGRAMS

Look for programs run by qualified individuals. The program should focus on teaching children and families how to improve eating habits. Stay away from programs that use quick weight loss methods.

Use the following checklist when choosing a weight management program for your child:

- Is the program staffed with a variety of health care professionals? The best programs use several professionals, including RDNs, exercise physiologists, pediatricians, and psychiatrists or psychologists.

- Does the program provide for an assessment from a qualified physician? Before your child starts a program, a doctor should check your child's weight and health. This exam should be explained to both you and the child.

- Does the program focus on changing behavior? The program should help change family behavior. It should teach hunger awareness. It should help pick out environmental factors related to eating. It should teach your child to stop thinking about foods as good or bad. And it should help children learn how to identify, express, and deal with feelings.

- Does the program avoid focusing on a specific diet? The program should teach your child how to select from a variety of healthy foods in portions that are right for your child.

- Does the program encourage daily activity and regular exercise? The program should help your child to be active.

- Are parents expected to be a key part of the program? You need to be involved in the program for it to work.

HEALTH CARE PROFESSIONALS AND RESOURCES

If you need to find a doctor for your child, look for one who specializes in childhood weight management. The American Academy of Pediatrics (AAP) can help you find one. Contact AAP at 708/228-5005 or www.aap.org.

An RDN can help too. Your doctor or pediatrician may be able to refer you or you can find an RDN through the Academy of Nutrition and Dietetics' "Find an Expert" online referral service at www.eatright.org.

A family counselor may help if you find it difficult to make family changes. Look for a psychologist or psychotherapist with an MA, MS, MSW, PhD, or psychology degree. Often, these counselors specialize in family counseling or eating disorders.

Cookbooks

Patti B. Geil and Tami A. Ross. *Cooking Up Fun for Kids with Diabetes.* Alexandria, VA: American Diabetes Association; 2003.

Nicola Graimes. *Kids' Fun and Healthy Cookbook.* London: DK Children; 2007.

Sally Sampson. *ChopChop: The Kids' Guide to Cooking Real Food with Your Family.* New York: Simon & Schuster; 2013.

Liz Weiss and Janice Newell Bissex. *No Whine with Dinner: 150 Healthy Kid-Tested Recipes from the Meal Makeover Moms.* Nashville, TN: Favorite Recipes Press; 2011.

Elisa Zied. *Feed Your Family Right: How to Make Smart Food and Fitness Choices for a Healthy Lifestyle.* New York: Wiley; 2007.

Books for Parents

Nimali Fernando and Potock, Melanie. *Raising a Healthy, Happy Eater: A Parent's Handbook: A Stage-by-Stage Guide to Setting Your Child on the Path to Adventurous Eating*. New York: The Experiment; 2015.

David Ludwig. *Ending the Food Fight: Guide Your Child to a Healthy Weight in a Fast Food/Fake Food World*. Boston, MA: Houghton Mifflin Harcourt, 2008.

Naomi Neufeld. *Kid Shape: A Practical Prescription for Raising Healthy, Fit Children*. Nashville, TN: Rutledge Hill Press; 2004.

Ellyn Satter. *Your Child's Weight: Helping Without Harming*. Madison, WI: Kelcy Press; 2005.

Ellyn Satter. *Secrets of Feeding a Healthy Family: How to Eat, How to Raise Good Eaters, How to Cook , 2nd ed*. Madison, WI: Kelcy Press; 2008.

Jodie Shield and Mary Mullen. *Healthy Eating, Healthy Weight for Kids and Teens*. Chicago, IL: Eatright Press; 2012.

Websites

Academy of Nutrition and Dietetics
www.eatright.org

American Council on Exercise
www.acefitness.org

American Academy of Pediatrics
www.healthychildren.org

We Can! Ways to Enhance Children's Activity & Nutrition
http://www.nhlbi.nih.gov/health/educational/wecan/

MyPlate
www.choosemyplate.gov

President's Council on Physical Fitness and Sports
www.fitness.gov

KidsHealth
www.kidshealth.org

KidsEatRight
www.kidseatright.org